Bruno Curiel

Skeletal and Dental response to long-term Herbst Appliance treatment

Bruno Curiel

Skeletal and Dental response to long-term Herbst Appliance treatment

A Cephalometric and CT scanning assessment

LAP LAMBERT Academic Publishing

Impressum / Imprint
Bibliografische Information der Deutschen Nationalbibliothek: Die Deutsche Nationalbibliothek verzeichnet diese Publikation in der Deutschen Nationalbibliografie; detaillierte bibliografische Daten sind im Internet über http://dnb.d-nb.de abrufbar.
Alle in diesem Buch genannten Marken und Produktnamen unterliegen warenzeichen-, marken- oder patentrechtlichem Schutz bzw. sind Warenzeichen oder eingetragene Warenzeichen der jeweiligen Inhaber. Die Wiedergabe von Marken, Produktnamen, Gebrauchsnamen, Handelsnamen, Warenbezeichnungen u.s.w. in diesem Werk berechtigt auch ohne besondere Kennzeichnung nicht zu der Annahme, dass solche Namen im Sinne der Warenzeichen- und Markenschutzgesetzgebung als frei zu betrachten wären und daher von jedermann benutzt werden dürften.

Bibliographic information published by the Deutsche Nationalbibliothek: The Deutsche Nationalbibliothek lists this publication in the Deutsche Nationalbibliografie; detailed bibliographic data are available in the Internet at http://dnb.d-nb.de.
Any brand names and product names mentioned in this book are subject to trademark, brand or patent protection and are trademarks or registered trademarks of their respective holders. The use of brand names, product names, common names, trade names, product descriptions etc. even without a particular marking in this work is in no way to be construed to mean that such names may be regarded as unrestricted in respect of trademark and brand protection legislation and could thus be used by anyone.

Coverbild / Cover image: www.ingimage.com

Verlag / Publisher:
LAP LAMBERT Academic Publishing
ist ein Imprint der / is a trademark of
OmniScriptum GmbH & Co. KG
Bahnhofstraße 28, 66111 Saarbrücken, Deutschland / Germany
Email: info@lap-publishing.com

Herstellung: siehe letzte Seite /
Printed at: see last page
ISBN: 978-3-659-82430-2

TABLE OF CONTENTS

SUMMARY The objectives of the study were to evaluate the skeletal and dental changes in the vertical and sagittal dimensions that occurred in the maxilla and in the mandible following a long-term Herbst Appliance treatment; and to assess any sagittal changes between the mandibular condyle and the glenoid fossa during Herbst therapy. The study sample consisted of 90 patients divided into treated and control groups. The 50 patients of the treated group had Class II Division 1 malocclusion and were 8.6 +/- 1.05 years old when treatment with a modified Herbst appliance was initiated. The Herbst appliance was used for a period of 20 months. The control untreated group was comprised of 40 patients, 9.7 +/- 1.08 years old with the same type of malocclusion. In the treated group, cephalographs were taken before cementing the appliance (T1), at the end of the Herbst phase treatment before debonding 20 months later (T2) and on average 2.8 years post-debonding (T3). In the control group these radiographs were taken before (T1) and after an examination period of 18 months (T2). Seven skeletal and 9 dental cephalometric measurements were analysed according to Pancherz method in all 90 subjects. Additionally, 18 treated cases had CT radiographs before bonding of the appliance (T1) and at the end of the Herbst treatment (20 months later) prior to debonding (T2). Condylar position changes induced by the appliance were analysed at the anterior and posterior joint spaces following Kamelchuck et al. method. Statistical comparison between treated and control groups for all parameters at T1 and T2 was performed with ANOVA with repeated measures. T-test analysis examined the Joint Space Index between T1 and T2 of the CT radiographs. Correlation between skeletal and dental parameters in the treated group and between skeletal and dental parameters in the control group was undertaken with Pearson's correlation test.

As a consequence of the Herbst therapy, in the treated group the maxillary sagittal anterior growth (A-OLp) was found to be significantly restrained while the mandibular skeletal sagittal parameter (Pog to OLp) significantly increased as compared with the control group.

In the treated group, the growth trend of mesial drift of the upper molar was limited while the lower incisor and the lower molar were displaced forward significantly compared to the control group from T1 to T2.

A substantial increase was found in the distance Co-Pog, which increased considerably from T1 to T2 from 99.98±4.47 mm to 104.44±4.79 mm in group 1. In comparison with previous studies, it was found in the treated group that the correction in the Class II was achieved mainly by effect on the mandibular corpus with less maxillary dental movement. As a result, the proper goal of the functional appliance by advancing the mandible was more concerned while the stability as a consequence of the movement created, was increased.

These main differences could take place as the force delivered by the Herbst appliance was better controlled as it was produced over a longer range of time.

3

INTRODUCTION

One of the most frequent problems presented to the orthodontist concerns the correction of skeletal Class II malocclusions. In many cases, the improper malocclusion is caused by the lower jaw that is posteriorly positioned in relationship to the rest of the face.

Improving patient's facial profile and normalizing the occlusion by reducing mandibular retrognathism and producing orthognathic relationship are the general objectives in correcting a skeletal Class II malocclusion.

When the patient is still growing it is possible to accentuate the growth of the mandible to catch up the upper part of the face by using fixed or removable functional appliances that propels the mandible in a protruded position during treatment. The use of functional appliance remained controversial[1] because previous studies have shown varying degrees of success in the treatment outcomes.[2]

One of the most popular fixed functional appliances used today is the Herbst bite jumping appliance[3] which produces a combine effect including inhibition of maxillary growth and stimulation of mandibular growth to achieve Class I skeletal relationships.[4] The Herbst Appliance is a fixed bite jumping device which does not require any cooperation from the patient, affects 24 hours a day and is generally used for a short treatment time approximately 6 to 8 months.[3]

The appliance was originally introduced by Emil Herbst, at the International Dental Congress in Berlin in 1905. In 1934 Herbst presented a series of articles in the Zahnärztliche Rundschau on his experiences with the appliance.[5] After 1934, however, very little was published on the subject, and the treatment method was more or less forgotten.

About 40 years later, Pancherz[6] called attention to the possibilities of stimulating mandibular growth by means of the Herbst appliance. In subsequent articles the effects of the appliance on the dentofacial complex[7-10] and on the masticatory system were evaluated. Recently the Herbst treatment method has gained increasing interest, especially in the United States, and several articles on appliance design have been published.[11]

Most articles about Herbst appliance therapy have been published by Pancherz[8] who measured mandibular length as the distance between condylion and gnathion on cephalograms taken with open mouth. Pancherz found skeletal correction by way of condylar growth stimulation utilizing the Herbst appliance over a period of 7 months. However, while some authors state that the skeletal effect of functional therapy is confined to maxillary growth restriction[12], others are of the opinion that functional therapy stimulates condylar growth as well as bone apposition in the glenoid fossa.[13]

According to Aelbers14, among various type of functional appliances, only the Herbst therapy is able to change mandibular growth up to a clinical significant extent. Clear radiological evidence of "fossa-remodelling" could not be established, and histologic changes of the glenoid fossa in animal studies seem to support this hypothesis.[15]

Actually, the mechanisms of TMJ response to "jumping of the bite" with the Herbst appliance are still unclear: on TMJ radiographs double contours of the anterior surface of the post-glenoid spine have been demonstrated in some patients, indicating bone remodelling.[16] However, cephalometric radiographs demonstrated an insignificant post-treatment anterior condylar position[17]. Using computed tomography (CT) double contours could be identified on the postero-superior part of the condyle and the glenoid fossa in single subjects by Paulsen et al.[18]

More recently, Paulsen and Karle[19] analyzed the temporomandibular joints changes using CT scanning and orthopantomograms but only on two subjects. Thus, the mechanism by which the temporomandibular joint (TMJ) responds to functional appliance therapy is still a matter of controversy.[15, 20]

Lately, Popowich et al[21] searched among all publications since 1966 to 2001 that were evaluating the effect of Herbst appliance therapy on temporomandibular joint (TMJ) morphology. Evidence of osseous remodeling or condyle position change could not be concluded and methodological deficiencies prevented major conclusions regarding disc position. Finally, they highlighted the importance of further research.

Since all studies using the Herbst appliance have been conducted over a similar short period of treatment (6-8 months) the duration of the treatment might be a crucial factor in the success of such treatment. Therefore the treatment time used in this study will be increased to 20 months.

OBJECTIVES

The objectives of the study were:

1. To evaluate the skeletal and dental changes both in the vertical and sagittal dimensions that occured in the maxilla and in the mandible after a long-term treatment with the Herbst appliance.

2. To assess the stability of the treatment results.

3. To assess any correlation between the different parameters.

4. To assess any sagittal changes between the mandibular condyle and the glenoid fossa during Herbst treatment.

HYPOTHESIS

1- The change over time in skeletal and dental parameters will differ between the treated and control groups a – The increase in dento-skeletal mandibular parameters will be greater in the treated than the control group.

b – The increase in dento-skeletal maxillary parameters will be smaller in the treated than the control group.

2. The results achieved by the Herbst appliance are stable during time.

3- There is no effect of the Herbst appliance on the position of the condyle relative to the glenoid fossa.

MATERIAL AND METHODS

Subjects

The sample consisted of 90 patients divided into:

- A treated group comprised of 50 consecutive Class II Division 1 malocclusion patients (25 boys and 25 girls) treated with a modified Herbst appliance during a time period of 20 months.
The patients had an overjet of at least 6 mm and were in the mixed dentition meaning that at least all four first permanent molars and all maxillary and mandibular incisors had erupted. The age at the start of treatment was 8.6±1.05 years old. The patients were all of white ethnicity, European type. This sample was selected from patients treated by the same practitioner and with the same appliance. Initially, none of the patients had any TMJ symptoms or contraindications for taking CT radiographs.

- A control group comprised of 40 subjects (19 boys and 21 girls) with a mean age 9.7±1.08 years old and with the same type of malocclusion and skeletal morphology as the treated group. The control group was followed up with no treatment during a time period of 18 months.

7

Appliance design

The Herbst appliance is a fixed functional appliance working as an artificial joint between the maxilla and the mandible (Fig.1, 2). A telescope mechanism on either side of the jaw, attached to orthodontics bands, keeps the mandible continuously in an anterior advanced position during all mandibular functions. The telescope tube is attached to the maxillary permanent first molar band and the telescope plunger to the mandibular first premolar band.[11]

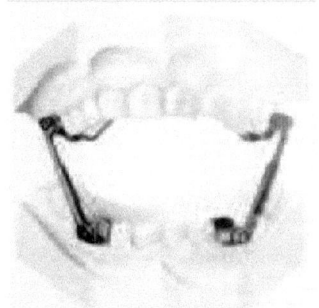 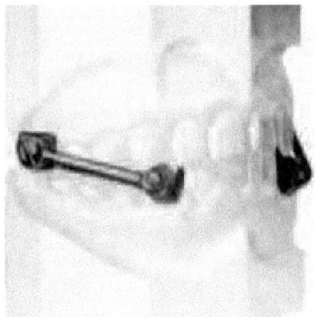

Fig 1: Herbst appliance (mouth opened)   Fig 2: Herbst appliance (mouth closed)

The Pruvost's modified Herbst appliance[22] (Fig.3) is made of casted crowns[23] replacing the regular prefabricated bands and it covers generally the first permanent molar and the deciduous molars in both upper and lower dentitions. Both sides of the lower part of the appliance are connected with a casted lingual and labial bar covering the lower incisors which enhances the rigidity and adaptability.

The modified Herbst appliance[22] is made from Nickel Chromium material and no coverage on the occlusal surfaces of posterior teeth is required.

At the start of treatment, the mandible is advanced anteriorly to an edge-to-edge position between the central incisors, thus placing the dental arches in a Class I or overcorrected Class I relationship with the posterior teeth out of occlusion. The anterior edge-to-edge position is reached progressively with a step by step mandibular advancement, depending on the severity of the malocclusion.

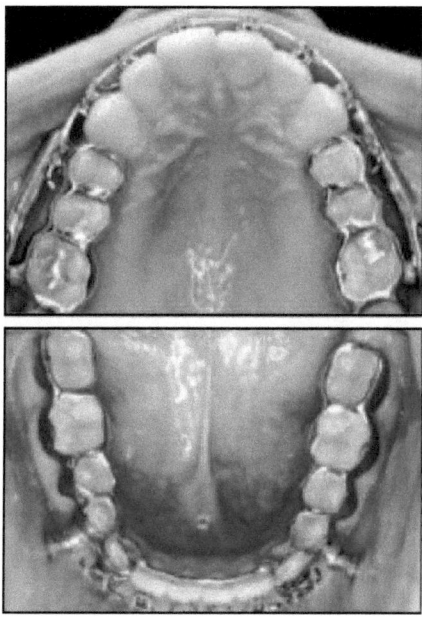

Fig 3: The Pruvost's Modified Herbst Appliance

Analysis of lateral radiographs

Sagittal and vertical skeletal and dental relationships occurring during the examination period were analysed by means of two lateral radiographs – one in centric occlusion and one with the mouth wide open. The latter cephalograph was used to visualize precisely the mandibular condyle, thus leading to a precise measure of the distance Condylion-Pogonion.

In the treated group, cephalographs were taken before cementing the appliance (T1), before debonding the appliance 20 months later (T2), and finally at a latter time point on average 2.8 years (T3) after T1.

In the control group, lateral radiographs were taken at T1 and after a follow up period of 18 months (T2).

The cephalographs were traced on matte acetate tracing film. Linear measurements were made to the nearest 0.5 mm.

The cephalometric analysis was based on 7 skeletal and 9 dental measurements analyzed according to Pancherz method[8] (Figs 4,5).

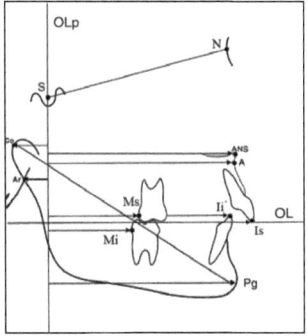 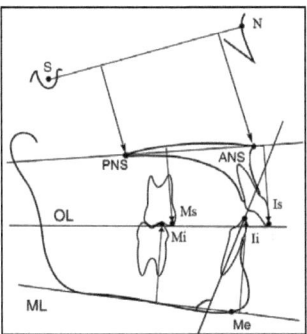

Fig 4: Horizontal measurements   Fig 5: Vertical measurements

Measuring procedure

The following lines were traced:

OL (occlusal line) — A line through the incisal edge of the upper central incisor (Is) and the distobuccal cusp of the maxillary permanent first molar.

OLp (occlusal line perpendiculare) — A line perpendicular to OL through Sella point (S).

For all linear measurements, the occlusal line (OL) and the occlusal line perpendicular (OLp) from the first head film (T1) were used as a reference grid. This grid was then transferred from the first tracing to the following tracings (T2, T3) by superimposition of the tracings on the Nasion-Sella line (NSL) with Sella (S) serving as a fixed reference point[4]. All registrations were done parallel to OL and perpendicular to OLp.

The lateral radiograph analysis included the following variables:

Skeletal measurements

A-OLp — Position of the maxillary base expressed by the distance from A point to OLp line.

Pog-OLp — Position of the mandibular base expressed by the distance from Pogonion to OLp line.

Co-OLp — Position of the condylar head expressed by the distance from Condylon to OLp line.

Co-Pog — Mandibular length (Condylion - Pogonion).

Mp-SN — Angle between Sella-Nasion and Mandibular Plane.

ANS-OLp — Position of the maxillary base expressed by the distance from Anterior Nasal Spine to OLp line.

ANS-Me — Lower anterior facial height expressed by the distance from Anterior Nasal Spine to Menton.

Dental measurements

Is-OLp — Position of the maxillary central incisor in the sagittal plane given by the distance from the tip of the upper central incisor to the OLp line.

Ii-OLp — Position of the mandibular central incisor in the sagittal plane given by the distance from the tip of the lower central incisor to the OLp line.

Ms-OLp — Position of the maxillary permanent first molar in the sagittal plane given by the distance from the distal cusp of the upper first molar to the OLp line.

Mi-OLp — Position of the mandibular permanent first molar in the sagittal plane given by the distance from the distal cusp of the lower first molar to the OLp line.

Is-Mx — Position of the maxillary central incisor in the vertical plane given by the distance from the tip of the upper central incisor to the maxillary plane (ANS-PNS).

Ms-Mx — Position of the maxillary permanent first molar in the vertical plane given by the distance from the mesial cusp of the upper first molar to the maxillary plane (ANS-PNS).

Ii-Mp — Position of the mandibular central incisor in the vertical plane given by the distance from the tip of the lower central incisor to the mandibular plane.

Mi-Mp — Position of the mandibular permanent first molar in the vertical plane given by the distance from the mesial cusp of the lower first molar to the mandibular plane.

Mp-Ii — Axial inclination of mandibular incisor (in degrees) to the mandibular plane.

Is-OLp minus Ii-Olp : Overjet.
Ms-OLp minus Mi-OLp : Molar relationship (a positive value indicates a distal molar relationship (Class II); a negative value indicates a normal molar relationship (Class I) or a mesial molar relationship (Class III).

CT scan evaluation: Analysis of temporomandibular joints (TMJ)

Treatment effect on the TMJ was assessed by CT scanning using a machine called "High Speed General Electric" which provides helical aquisitions; it allowed an aquisition of the whole volume required and then restituted in slices through a software called "Dentascan". Adaptating the size of the image aquisition and its restitution, the computer program provided each slice in a ratio 1:1 (no magnification). While the patient laid down on one's back with the head straight, the software program made any required correction if any change of the head position occurred.

Eighteen treated patients from the treated sample had CT radiographs before bonding of the appliance (T1) and at the end of the Herbst treatment (20 months later) prior to debonding (T2). For ethical reasons, we did not perform CT scan in the control group with no treatment justification.

Condylar position changes induced by the appliance were analysed at the anterior and posterior joint spaces in the sagittal plane. For each left and right TMJ, CT scans were performed by means of millimetric slices with the mouth closed; the central section which crossed the condyle in its center was selected for the analysis. This slice was scanned and magnified 5 folds and the distances were calculated with computed software, "Adobe Photoshop". The CT of both the left and the right TMJ from before (T1) and after (T2) Herbst treatment were traced and analysed according to the method described by Kamelchuck et al (Fig 6).[24]

To eliminate the problem of differences in joint sizes when comparing the individuals, a Joint Space Index was calculated:

Joint Space Index = [(Post – Ant) / (Post + Ant)] x 100

Where Post is the posterior joint space and Ant is the anterior joint space.

The intersection between the tangent from the most superior point of the fossa (X point) to the outer curve of the condyle gave one point. The posterior joint space was defined as the distance from this tangent to the glenoid fossa.

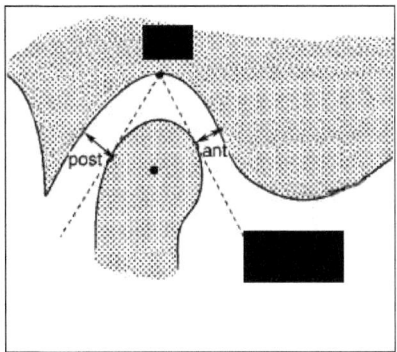

Fig 6 : assessment of the position of the condyle

A Joint-Space-Index of '0' value indicated a centric condylar position; a negative Joint-Space-Index indicated a posterior condylar position and a positive an anterior condylar position.

For exemple, if the posterior distance equals 2 as well as the anterior one, then the index is:
JSI = [(2 – 2) / (2 + 2)] x 100 = (0 / 4) x 100 = 0 x 100 = 0

Indeed, when the posterior distance equals the anterior distance, the condylar posture is centered in the glenoid fossa ie, equals to zero.

RESULTS

Cephalograms analysis

Mean differences between the cephalograms analysis were calculated for both groups (G1, G2) at T1, T2 and for the treated group (G1) at T3. Findings are displayed in Tables 1, 2, 3, 4 and 5.

Horizontal measurements

Maxilla
In the treated group (G1), the distance for both maxillary skeletal points, A and ANS to OLp increased with time but more considerably from T2 to T3 (1.32 ± 1.32 mm for A point and 1.12 ± 1.55 mm for ANS point) than from T1 to T2 (0.94 ± 0.67 mm for A point and 0.84 ± 0.78 mm for ANS point) when the appliance was worn. (Table 5)
Consequently, the maxillary sagittal anterior growth (A-OLp) was found to be significantly restrained in the treated group (0.94 ± 0.67 mm) compared with the control group (1.42 ± 1.16 mm) with a $p =0.023**$ (Table 4).

Mandible
On the contrary, in the treated group the mandibular skeletal sagittal parameter (Pog to OLp) also increased with time from T1 to T2 and from T2 to T3. (Table 1)
From T1 to T2, Pog-OLp in group 1 (3.26 ± 1.26 mm) differed significantly ($p<0.001$) from the control group (1.64 ± 1.31 mm) (Table 5); the net effect in group 1 was 1.62 mm greater than in the control group. (Table 4)

Maxillary dental arch
In the treated group, from T1 to T2, both upper molar and incisor kept nearly the same antero-posterior position (0.23 ± 1.15 mm and 0.35 ± 1.68 mm, respectively) (Table 4).
There was a significant increase in the upper molar position in the control group as compared to the treated group ($p<0.001$); the upper incisor distance increased more in the control group as compared to the treated group but this change was not significant ($p=0.063$) (Table 4). That is, the Herbst appliance in the treated group limited the growth trend of mesial drift of the upper molar.

Mandibular dental arch

In the treated group, the lower incisor moved forward significantly 4.61±1.59 mm and the lower molar about 4.39±1.38 mm from T1 to T2 (Table 4). From T2 to T3, these changes were of 0.87±2 mm for the lower incisor and 1.87±3.06 mm for the lower molar (table 5).

In the treated group, both the lower incisor and the lower molar were displaced forward significantly compared to the control group from T1 to T2.

The forward movement of the lower incisor was greater than that of the lower molar (4.61±1.59 mm and 4.39±1.38 mm, respectively). (Table 4)

In the treated group, the degree of proclination of the lower incisor to the mandibular plane increased from 97.05±5.88° to 99.03±6.05° from T1 to T2. (Table 3)

However, this change (1.98±2.64 mm) as compared to the control group (1.4±1.85 mm) was not significant (p=0.244) (Table 4). In the treated group, the proclination that appeared during the Herbst phase (99.03±6.05 mm at T2) remained the same (99.25±5.96 mm at T3) during the second stage of treatment with the fixed edgewise appliance. (Table 1)

Interjaw relationship

Long-term Herbst therapy resulted in significantly improved dental and skeletal relationships: in group 1, the overjet was decreased from 7.27±2.04 mm at T1 to 2.66±2.19 mm at T2 (Table 1) while in the control group, the overjet was decreased from 6.95±2.65 mm at T1 to 5.07±2.52 mm at T2. (Table 2)

At T2, the overjet was reduced by 1.87±1.22 mm in the control group but was significantly more reduced by 4.61±1.59 mm in the treated group (p <0.001). (Table 4)

The molar relationship had improved by approximately 4.16 mm in the treated group as compared to 0.83 mm in the control group. This difference was found to be highly significant (p <0.001). (Table 4)

Vertical measurements

Maxilla

In the treated group, the maxillary anterior skeletal vertical change (N-ANS) (Fig. 2) increased significantly from 45.66±3.04 mm to 47.92±2.92 mm from T1 to T2 (Table 1); the posterior part of the maxilla (measured by PNS-SN) was also significantly lowered but to a lesser extent (1.41±1.09 mm). (Table 4)

In the vertical plane, the inferior displacement of the upper molar was significantly smaller in the treated group (0.62±0.71 mm) as compared to the control group (1.6±0.95 mm) (p<0.001). (Table 4) That is, in relation to the control group, the upper molar in the treated group was intruded.

Mandible

In group 1, the mandibular plane angle (Mp-SN) increased from T1 to T2 from 32.96±4.86° to 33.62±4.98°. (Table 1) As it did not show any treatment effect, the anterior facial height increased in the same manner with no significant difference between the 2 groups.

In the mandible, the difference between groups concerning incisor extrusion was found to be significant (p = 0.007) from T1 to T2. That is the lower incisors were intruded in the treated group in comparison to the control. (Table 4)

Horizontal-vertical measurements

A substantial increase was found in the distance Co-Pog, which increased considerably from T1 to T2 from 99.98±4.47 mm to 104.44±4.79 mm in the group 1. (Table 1)

This increase in the length of the mandible was significantly higher in the treated group as compared to the control group (p<0.001); A displacement of 4.55±2.47 mm was measured in the treated group compared with only 1.6±1.04 mm for the control group from T1 to T2. (Table 4)

While the change from Pog to OLp was considerable in the treated group (3.26±1.26 mm), the horizontal change in Co to OLp was minute (0.43±0.9 mm) although significant (p = 0.008) (Table 4).
Also, Articulare point was basically not affected in the horizontal dimension by the treatment effects.

Condyle analysis of the treated group (G1)

Analysis by %:

As described previously, the Joint Space Index (Fig.3) is the ratio which was expressed in percentage for each left and right condyle per time point T1 or T2.
- If JSI is positive then the condyle is anteriorly positionned in the glenoid fossa
- If JSI is negative then the condyle is posteriorly positionned in the glenoid fossa
- If JSI = 0: the condyle is in the center of the glenoid fossa

The assessment of the position of the *left* condyle revealed:

At T1: (Table 7)
- A posterior position of the condyle in 11.8% of the group
- A neutral position in 23.5% of the group
- An anterior position in 64.7% of the group

At T2: (Table 9)

- Only 5.9% of the condyle remained posteriorly in the glenoid fossa
- 41.2% appeared to be centered
- 52.9% showed an anterior position

The assessment of the position of the *right* condyle revealed:

At T1: (Table 8)
- A posterior position in 29.4% of the group
- A neutral position in 17.7% of the group
- An anterior position in 52.9% of the group

At T2: (Table 10)
- 23.5% of the group remained posteriorly in the glenoid fossa
- 23.6% appeared to be centered
- 52.9 % showed an anterior position

Changes (Δ) in JSI from T1 to T2 (table 9 & 10):

ΔJSIL = JSI (t2) – JSI (t1) for the left condyle

ΔJSIR = JSI (t2) – JSI (t1) for the right condyle

- A positive ΔJSI indicates that an anterior displacement of the condyle with no remodeling of the glenoid fossa occurred at the end of the Herbst treatment.

- A negative or zero ΔJSI indicates that either the condyle did not move anteriorly initially, or that the Herbst treatment caused initiation of bone remodelling from T1 to T2.

Example:

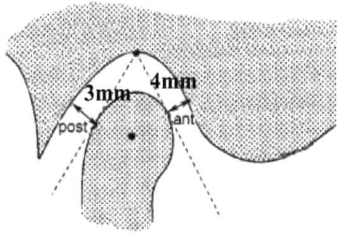
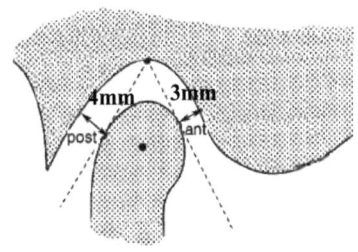

Position of the condyle T1   Position of the condyle T2

At T1 : JSI (t1) = (3-4) / (3+4) = -1/7 = - 14%

At T2 : JSI (t2) = (4-3) / (3+4) = +1/7 = +14%

ΔJSI = T2 – T1 = +28% ; this example showed that positive ΔJSI of +28% is due to 1 mm anterior displacement of the condyle with no bone apposition on the posterior wall of the glenoid fossa.

From T1 to T2, the difference in the joint space index was negative or equal to 0 in 47.1% of the cases, meaning that a remodelling probably took place (table 10). The cumulative percent showed that in 82.4%, ΔJSIL was less than 5.88 %; by considering the previous example where a ΔJSI of +28% represented a 1 mm anterior displacement of the condyle, it could be concluded that a ΔJSIL of less than 5.88 % represents an anterior movement of only 0.2 mm.

Therefore, in 82.2%, the condyle was displaced 0.2 mm anteriorly.

In 64.7% and 52.9% of the cases, the left and right condyles were anteriorly positioned before treatment, respectively. (Table 7 & 9).

After advancing the mandible at the end of the Herbst treatment phase (T2), the condyle resumed a more centered position in the glenoid fossa.

The difference in the joint space index (%) change was found to be not significant for each condyle from T1 to T2 (p = 0.422 for the right condyle change and p = 0.928 for the left one).

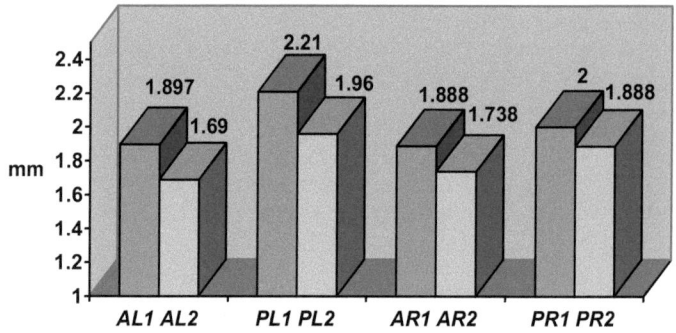

Graph 1: Mean value (mm) of the anterior (A) and posterior (P) position of the left (L) and right (R) condyle at T1 (blue) and T2 (yellow)

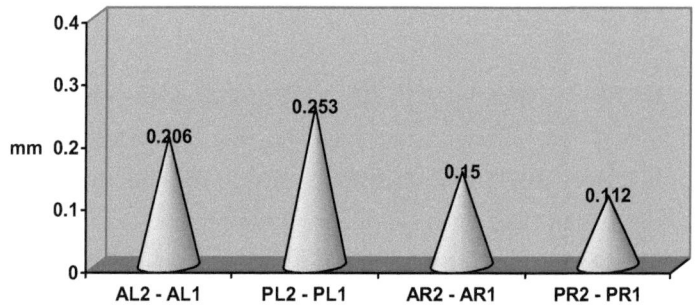

Graph 2: Difference in the position of the condyle between 2 times (T2 – T1)

Analysis by mm:

Concerning the left condyle, the distance between the condyle to the anterior border of the glenoid fossa decreased by 0.206 mm, meaning that the condyle was displaced forward (Graph 1 & Graph 2). The distance between the left condyle to the posterior border of the fossa also decreased by 0.253 mm.

In the anterior part of the fossa, where a compression may have been produced, resorption in the anterior part of the fossa and/or in the anterior part of the condyle may have occured. On the contrary, apposition may have taken place in the posterior part of the fossa and/or in the posterior part of the condyle.

Notice that the amount of apposition that was produced was greater than the amount of resorption.

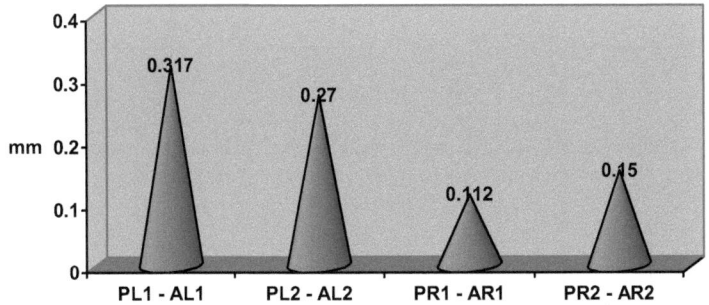

Graph 3: Assesment of the antero-posterior position of the condyle in the glenoid fossa at each time T1 and T2.

When comparing the left and right condyle, graph 3 showed that a bigger initial displacement was associated with more remodelling during treatment.

For example, for the right condyle:

The initial deplacement (PR1-AR1) was 0.112 mm (T1). The condyle was displaced anteriorly (AR2-AR1) by 0.150 mm. In theory and with no remodelling, PR2 should be equal to PR1 + 0.150 = 2.15mm;

But PR2 was 1.88 mm meaning that some remodelling by apposition probably took place. The amount of the remodelling was calculated by the difference between the theoretical PR2 and the practical PR2: 2.15 – 1.88 = 0.27 mm.

For the left condyle: by the same approach, we found a remodelling of 0.456 mm for an initial displacement of 0.206 mm.
Finally, it seemed that the amount of remodelling produced was proportionnal to the amount of displacement induced.

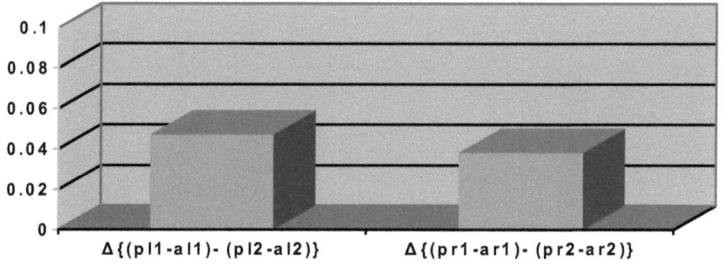

Table AB : The differences between the displacement achieved from T1 to T2.

For the left condyle, the anterior and the posterior displacement achieved from T1 to T2 were not significant (p=0.712). The same conclusion was found for the right condyle (p=0.637).

DISCUSSION

- T1 to T2 is the period of time where the appliance was inserted. The Herbst appliance which is bonded is supposed to deliver a continuous orthopedic effect as well as a dental effect.

In both groups, A and ANS to OLp increased; these distances expressed the horizontal growth of the maxilla which occured from T1 to T3. This maxillary sagittal anterior growth (A-OLp) was found to be significantly restrained compared with the control group and also with the time period from T2 to T3, where the growth potential of the maxilla could be fully expressed since no Herbst appliance was worn. This suggests that the Herbst appliance is delivering a distal force vector to the maxillary complex through the dentition, therefore exerting a growth restraining effect on the maxillary arch as found by Pangrazio-Kulbersh and Berger[25].

However, Croft et al.[26] reported a 1.2 mm restraint of the sagittal displacement of A point; by observing a posterior translation of A point at the end of treatment, they showed a complete restriction in the growth of the maxilla which could not be confirmed in the present study since A point moved anteriorly of 0.94±0.67 mm. (Table 4)

A first explanation may be related to the treatment duration; indeed, while using the Herbst for only 7 months, significant growth changes in the maxilla due to growth itself may not be sufficient to be expressed. This study observed the changes over a period of time of 2 years; with such a long-term duration, despite of the appliance effect, horizontal growth potential of the maxilla could be expressed and occured as confirmed by the increase in A and ANS to OLp.

Moreover, by extending the treatment time in our study, the force delivered by the appliance could be progressively and proportionally increased as the mandible was progressively advanced, thus delivering a more progressive amount of force on the upper dentition. Falck and

Fränkel[27] indicated that the restraining effect of these forces on the maxilla could be eliminated, or at least minimized, when the mandible was advanced in small steps of 2 mm; that is, because the retractors were only slightly stretched. In a group in which the initial construction bite was taken with the incisors in an end-to-end relationship, a significant restraining effect on maxillary basal development was recognizable; in another group with the step by step mandibular advancement, A point moved anteriorly.

The fact that the horizontal growth of the maxilla, was greater from T2 to T3 than from T1 to T2, suggests that the Herbst appliance did not prevent completely the forward growth of the maxilla but restrained it to a certain extent. This hypothesis is confirmed by comparing both treated and control groups together where more horizontal growth occurred in the control group with a significant difference.

Since the post-treatment period of the treated group (T2 to T3) was greater than the corresponding period in the control group (T1 to T2) more horizontal growth took place in the treated group than in the control group.

The same conclusion could be drawn for the distance measured from Pog to OLp which increased in the treated group continuously from T1 to T2 to T3.

In fact, from T1 to T2, the increase was 3.26±1.26 mm in the treated group while it was only of 1.64±1.31 mm for the control group. (Table 4) That is, a two-fold increase in the treated group as compared to the control group. This confirms the positive effect of the Herbst appliance which propelled the mandible in a forward position and finally acted as a potential stimulator of mandibular growth.

No Herbst appliance was worn in the treated group from T2 to T3 and the increase in Pog to OLp was still significant (1.75±1.7 mm). Producing more horizontal growth in the mandible than the control group, the only difference being the amount of time between these two measurements: in the treated group, we measured the growth that occurred from the age of 10.5 years for a mean period of 2.8 years (T2-T3), while the control group was observed from 9.7 until 11.7 years (T1-T2) for a mean period of 2 years. Actually, this period of time between 11 to 14 years old matched the pubertal peak of growth and this may explained the net increase in horizontal mandibular growth as seen in the treated group. As reported by Hansen et al[28] there was a notable tendency toward greater chin projection following Herbst therapy in the older peak (3.8 mm) and postpeak (4.5 mm) groups, suggesting less improvement in patients treated in the mixed dentition. However, these patients whom the mean age was 8 years at T1, could benefit from two different separate phases of stimulation of the mandibular growth. As shown by Pancherz and Hägg[29], somatic maturation had a significant influence on the mandibular skeletal and dental treatment response.

Pancherz[30] found less magnitude and often temporary maxillary orthopedic effect in older patients. In contrast, patients treated in the mixed dentition showed greater response and adaptabilty in comparison to the non-growing group. However, the question if extending the treatment duration in growing patient will increase the response was not yet addressed.

Furthermore, Valant and Sinclair[31] reported a distal driving effect on the upper dentition after treatment while the appliance was worn for a shorter period of time (between 7 to 11 months). By extending the treatment duration in our study, a step by step mandibular advancement could be performed applying slighter forces on the upper dentition, thus, allowing more adaptive response of the adjacent tissues.

The investigations of Graf[32] and Witt and Komposch[33] have shown that in the presence of a skeletal Class II relationship, when the mandible is anteriorly displaced by one millimeter, the forces of the stretched retractors are approximately 1 N (100 gm). Therefore, when the initial construction bite is taken with the mandible displaced forward by 6 to 7 mm, considerable forces are transmitted to the dentition wherever the appliance contacts the teeth, which inevitably results in a tooth-moving effect. This may be the reason why Mills[34] in a critique on a rather large number of investigations of "functional appliance therapy" came to the conclusion that the major changes produced by the activator or its derivates were found to be essentially dental in nature.

Pancherz[35] assessed the extent, and the interrelation between, skeletal and dental components that contributed to Class II relapse after Herbst treatment. His findings revealed that relapse in the overjet and sagittal molar relationship resulted mainly from posttreatment maxillary and mandibular dental changes. In particular, the maxillary incisors and molars moved significantly ($p < 0.05$) to a more anterior position in the relapsed group than in the stable group. In our study, by exerting less force on the upper dentition which was allowed by the step by step mandibular advancement, the Class II correction was minimally achieved by a distal driving of the upper dentition therefore most likely limiting the potential relapse observed by Pancherz. While mesial maxillary dental translation was inhibited by the appliance, the molar relation improved more by advancement of the lower dentition as well as mandibular corpus growth, stimulated by the functional appliance (Table 4 and 5).

The appliance design used in our study offered a full coverage of the whole lower dentition including the lower incisors which should prevent their proclination. However, still some proclination appeared but the difference with the control group was found to be not significant.

Pancherz[4] showed that the mandibular incisors proclined an average of 6.6° during 6 months of Herbst treatment and that the general position of the maxillary incisors was unaffected by treatment.

Compared to these studies where the appliance was used on a short period of time, we could observe that extending the treatment time to approximately 24 months did not cause more side effects as proclination (1.98±2.64° from T1 to T2).

The modified Herbst appliance used in the present study was covering the whole dentition including the anterior teeth, thus offering a full and maximal anchorage, and finally reducing the amount of proclination that was obtained with a regular Herbst appliance design.

Indeed, Obijou and Pancherz[36] reported an anterior movement of the lower dentition (3.4±2.5 mm) with a significant proclination of the lower incisors (p < 0.05). In our treated group, the patients were treated in the early mixed dentition which offered more teeth as anchorage compared to a transitionnal dentition period where the deciduous molars might be missing.

In a previous investigation of Pancherz and Hansen[37], a difference between partial and total (incorporating more dental units) anchorage was confirmed for maxillary incisors and mandibular molars only: the upper front teeth were moved more lingually, and the lower molars were moved more mesially in the total than in the partial anchorage cases (p < 0.05). More recently, 3 different types of anchorage were compared between mandibular banded and cast splint anchorage forms used in Herbst treatment[38]; As the design of the Herbst appliance for the 3 types was not covering the anteriors and the therapy was conducted over a short period of 7 months, they concluded that none of the three mandibular anchorage forms used in Herbst treatment could prevent an anchorage loss, especially in the anterior region.

As seen in the treated group of the present study, the distance from a dental point to OLp increased more than the distance from a skeletal point to OLp. For example, the lower incisor was displaced from T1 to T2 about 4.61±1.59 mm as Pog was displaced about 3.26±1.26 mm. (Table 3) This is in agreement with Pancherz[23], who found that 60% of the Class II correction were achieved dentally and 40% skeletally. Using the Herbst appliance over a short period of time of 7 months, the overjet and molar relationships were corrected by different types of movement.

Konik et al[39] reported a molar correction to Class I of 6.1 mm which was due to 37% skeletal and 63% dental changes. The overjet correction of 8.4 mm was due to 27 % skeletal and 73% dental changes.

Therefore, it confirmed the idea whether the Herbst appliance is also a dental borne appliance.

We found that the intermolar functional correction was accomplished 75% by a mandibular skeletal advancement and 25% by mesial drift of lower molars. The maxillary changes did not contribute to the correction since no distal effect was produced but rather a restraining effect, which prevented deterioration of the intermolar relationship.

Also, Pancherz[36] reported a molar correction of 3.2 mm comprised of a distal movement of the upper molar of 1.6 mm and a forward movement of the lower molar of the same amount. He showed more maxillary restraint but less mandibular skeletal involvement. On the other hand, Falck and Fränkel[27] proved that treatment with a functional appliance in a group in which the initial construction bite was taken with the incisors in an end-to-end relationship had mainly a tooth-moving effect, whereas in his second group with a progressive step-by-step mandibular advancement, basal development of the mandible was stimulated sagittally. Finally, the extension in the treatment duration which allowed a more progressive mandibular advancement appeared to be a key factor in the correction of skeletal Class II with mandibular deficiency.

The Herbst appliance was delivering a force with a distal and vertical component of forces. The design of the appliance allowed a better distribution of the forces in the mandible compared to the maxilla. In the maxilla, the forces were principally directed to the first molars, in the vertical dimension.

These forces by acting on dental elements had probably an influence of the maxillary bone itself. Pancherz and Anehus-Pancherz[40] showed that the palatal plane tipped downward by 0.2° during Herbst treatment period. In comparison with the untreated Class II control group of their study, no significant difference was seen. Following Herbst direction of forces to the upper dentition, a downward tilting of the occlusal plane anteriorly occurred. The changes in the distance between N-ANS (1.86±1.27 mm) and PNS-SN (1.41±1 mm) lead to the change in the maxillary plane downward and forward as it was described previously. The appliance limited the normal development (extrusion) of the molars during growth. PNS was lowered more than the molar was extruded.

As a consequence, the molars were intruded relative to the normal vertical development of the maxilla. (Table 3)

In the vertical dimension, the mandibular plane angle to SN was unchanged as shown by previous studies. Croft et al[26] reported only a slight opening of the bite (0.6 mm); Ruf and Pancherz[41] showed that the mandibular plane angle was unaffected by Herbst therapy. In their study, a continuous decrease in the Mp-SN took place, posttreatment.

In contrast to the results of Valant and Sinclair[31], Herbst appliance therapy did not have a significant effect on the Mp-NS angle, as the initial opening was compensated during the active treatment and the settling period after treatment. Even though Mp-NS angle was almost unaffected by Herbst therapy (T1 to T2), continuous Mp-NS angle decrease took place during the follow-up period (T2 to T3) in almost all subjects, which could be interpreted as a result of a normalized function that permitted normal growth and development.

While the anterior facial height increased (T1-T3) we can assume that a compensating remodelling of the posterior part of the mandible occurred, either in the mandibular angle or in the condyle area causing no change in the Mp-NS angle. (Table 1)

The correlations matrix (Table 6) gave some indication as to the mechanism of functional correction. Therefore, regarding the relation between the change found in one parameter (skeletal or dental, horizontal or vertical, maxillary or mandibular parameters) to the change found in another parameter, we found that 12 of the 171 pairs of parameters were correlated significantly with 11 pairs being either of maxillary-versus-mandibular or maxillary-versus-maxillary. That is, 91.6% of the 12 pairs were related to maxillary parameters (Table 6). Also, 10 pairs were combined either of dental-versus-skeletal or skeletal-versus-skeletal meaning that 83.3% of the same 12 pairs were related to skeletal parameters. As found in Vardimon's article[42], this suggested that the skeletal parameters were regulating factors that controlled the functional correction process.

Mandibular length was usually expressed as the distance between Condylion (Co) and Pogonion (Pog). One of the problems encountered with this assessment is the difficulty in defining the head of the condyle on a cephalogram. Adenwalla[43] claimed that, if the mandibular condyle had to be used as an important landmark in any cephalometric study, the open mouth cephalogram should be taken and superimposed on the respective cephalogram in habitual occlusion, to obtain the most accurate and reliable measurements. For this reason the present radiographic cephalograms were taken with the mouth open which allowed an excellent visualization of the head of the condyle, therefore allowing a perfect measurement of the distance Co-Pog.

Pancherz[37] revealed that effective condylar growth could be increased during the Herbst treatment period of time. Our study confirmed these findings with a significant increase as compared to the control group. While the change from Pog to OLp was considerable in the treated group (3.26±1.26 mm) as compared to the control group (1.64±1.31 mm), the horizontal change in Co to OLp was minute (0.43±0.9 mm) although significant (p = 0.008) (Table 4).

Fischer[44] showed that the increased amount of condylar growth occurred in a posterior-superior direction. Condylar growth and "effective" TMJ changes were directed more vertically compared with the treatment changes.[45]
As measured in the horizontal dimension only, Vardimon et al[42] found a similar change in Ar between the treated group (0.67±1.29 mm) and the control group (0.28±0.59 mm).

In the TMJ area, Kohlas and Ruf[46] found anterior position of the condyles prior to treatment. However, the average condyle position was insignificantly more anterior post-treatment than pre-treatment.
Because glenoid fossa remodelling could only be vizualised at a later treatment stage (7 months) than condylar remodelling (3 months) [46], they could not assess changes in the fossa-condyle relationship when short-term Herbst appliance treatment was used.

Leaving the appliance for 24 months allowed full expression of the adaptive processes of the temporal bone (periosteal ossification) and the condyle (endochondral ossification). After advancing the mandible at the end of the Herbst treatment phase, the condyle was shown to be more centered in relation to its glenoid fossa. Our findings indicate that condylar and glenoid fossa remodelling as well as condyle-fossa relationship contributed to the increase in mandibular prognathism after a long period of Herbst appliance treatment.

Different theories attempted to explain how the condylar cartilage responded to an altered functional position of the condyle [47, 48, 49].
McNamara et al[50] showed an adaptive response in the form of hyperplasia of the prechondroblastic-chondroblastic area of the posterior and posterio-

superior border of the condyle after forward repositionning of the mandible.

As the condyle was displaced anteriorly, the anterior distance between the condyle to the fossa should have decreased. We also expected to see an increase in the posterior area between the condyle and the fossa at T2. However, this distance also decreased suggesting that a remodelling probably appeared in the relation of the condyle to its fossa (T2). (Graph 1 & Graph 2)

These findings are in agreements with Pancherz[45], who found after 6 to 12 weeks of therapy a partial relocation of the condyles in the fossa while they were displaced anteriorly out of the glenoid fossa and became positioned on the top of the articular eminence just after the initial bonding of the appliance.

They showed in the postero-superior region of the condyle a distinct area of increased signal intensity (bright areas) immediately below the signal-poor zone (dark areas) surrounding the condyle.

Paulsen[17] showed on CT scanning taken after Herbst insertion that new bone formation was revealed as double contours in the fossa articularis and at the posterior part of the condyle. Although we could not identify his radiographic findings, our measurements suggest that such changes took place.

Animal studies have shown that the temporal bone of the glenoid fossa adapts to protrusive function[51] with bone formation along the anterior border and bone resorption on the posterior border. Also Güner[52] tried to show that increased bone formation in the TMJs was analysed with the aid of pre- and post-treatment scintigraphic studies.

It could have been interesting to follow the evolution of the condyle on a long term and assess if the amount of resorption would finally be equal to the amount of apposition.

CONCLUSION

The use of an appliance that relocates the mandible anteriorly not only influences the effect of treatment upon the maxilla but may also affect mandibular growth and position, as demonstrated in mixed-dentition treatment.

There is reason to believe that there is a certain correlation between the amount of force and the orthopedic effect of treatment.

Extending the treatment duration to 20 months may appeared to be a key factor as it allowed a better control of the force delivered on both dentition; consequently and in comparison to previous studies with a shorter treatment time, the correction of the Class II was here achieved by :

- less effect on the maxilla, more effect on the mandible
- less dental effect, more skeletal effect
- less posterior maxillary dental translation and therefore less relapse potential

It is important to use the total dentoalveolar area in both the maxillary and the mandibular arches as anchorage for transferring forces to affect the interrelationship between maxillary and mandibular basal bones as well as the dental response to orthopedic forces.

Stimulation effect of the Herbst appliance on sagittal condylar growth, glenoid fossa remodelling and repositioning of the condyle within the fossa may explained the effective TMJ growth changes.

As a further research, it should be most interesting to analyze the effects of the extent on the treatment duration over the muscle activity, responsible of so many failures in orthodontics.

	Group 1 (treated group)					
Parameters	T1	T2	T3	P(t1-t2)	P(t2-t3)	P(t1-t3)
A- OLP (mm)	70.85±3.25	71.79±3.35	74.15±3.49	<0.001***	<0.001***	<0.001***
ANS-OLP (mm)	73.51±3.35	74.35±3.35	76.9±3.37	<0.001***	0.004**	<0.001***
Pog- OLP (mm)	69.77±4.74	73.03±4.59	76.37±6.3	<0.001***	<0.001***	<0.001***
Is- OLP (mm)	74.4±5.15	74.75±5.39	78.13±7.11	0.148	0.251	0.085
Ii- OLP (mm)	67.13±5.62	71.74±5.5	75.62±7.05	<0.001***	0.065	<0.001***
Ms- OLP (mm)	34.92±3.69	35.15±3.89	37.32±5.84	0.0163	0.002**	0.004**
Mi- OLP (mm)	33.11±3.71	37.5±3.86	39.65±5.89	<0.001***	0.013*	<0.001***
Co- OLP (mm)	10.98±2.53	11.41±2.44	11.15±2.77	0.001**	0.061	0.027*
Ar- OLP (mm)	7.23±2.26	7.82±2.13	8.62±2.61	<0.001***	0.278	0.001**
Mp- Ii (mm)	36.14±3.29	37.08±2.83	37±3.29	<0.001***	0.005**	<0.001***
Mp-Mi (mm)	27.51±2.87	28.62±2.75	28.45±3.1	0.251	0.085	<0.001***
Mp- Ii (°)	97.05±5.88	99.03±6.05	99.25±5.96	<0.001***	0.947	0.013**
Mp- Sn (°)	32.96±4.86	33.62±4.98	33.02±4.64	0.005**	0.793	0.044*
Mx- Is (mm)	26.01±2.82	27.97±2.84	27.9±2.82	<0.001***	0.012*	<0.001***
Mx- Ms (mm)	17.5±2.9	18.12±2.84	18.55±2.07	<0.001***	0.001**	<0.001***
Na- ANS (mm)	45.66±3.04	47.92±2.92	49.87±3.72	<0.001***	0.018*	<0.001***
SN- PNS (mm)	38.88±2.97	40.29±2.88	41.97±3.12	<0.001***	0.029*	<0.001***
ANS- Me (mm)	58.08±3.79	59.97±3.75	62.22±4.69	<0.001***	0.004**	<0.001***
Co- Pog (mm)	99.89±4.47	104.44±4.79	109.225±7.59	<0.001***	<0.001***	<0.001***
Overjet (mm)	7.27±2.04	2.66±2.19		<0.001***		

Table 1 : Comparison between 3 different time point T1, T2, T3 for group G1 (treated group)

Parameters	Group 2 (control group)		
	T1	T2	P
A- OLP (mm)	73.57 ± 5.82	75 ± 5.89	<0.001***
ANS-OLP(mm)	76.37 ± 6.27	77.98 ± 6.27	<0.001***
Pog- OLP (mm)	73.12 ± 7.45	74.76 ± 7.62	<0.001***
Is- OLP (mm)	80.35 ± 6.87	81.53 ± 6.85	0.005**
Ii- OLP (mm)	73.4 ± 7.1	75.27 ± 7	<0.001***
Ms- OLP (mm)	37.75 ± 5.05	39.78 ± 5.32	<0.001***
Mi- OLP (mm)	36.25 ± 5.57	39.11 ± 5.43	<0.001***
Co- OLP (mm)	11.71 ± 3.06	11.53 ± 3.31	0.373
Ar- OLP (mm)	8.18 ± 3.17	8.18 ± 3.39	1.00
Mp- Ii (mm)	36.27 ± 3.54	37.86 ± 3.43	<0.001***
Mp-Mi (mm)	27.55 ± 2.91	28.33 ± 3.53	0.006*
Mp- Ii (°)	96.38 ± 7.54	97.78 ± 7.38	<0.001***
Mp- Sn (°)	33.48 ± 5.55	33.36 ± 5.61	0.531
Mx- Is (mm)	25.58 ± 3.32	27.19 ± 3.12	<0.001***
Mx- Ms (mm)	17.68 ± 2.04	19.28 ± 2.4	<0.001***
Na- ANS (mm)	47.17 ± 3.63	48.37 ± 3.8	<0.001***
SN- PNS (mm)	39.92 ± 3.35	40.5 ± 3.35	<0.001***
ANS- Me (mm)	60.23 ± 4.9	61.72 ± 4.84	<0.001***
Co- Pog (mm)	101.63 ± 6.32	103.23 ± 6.28	<0.001***
Overjet (mm)	6.95 ±2.65	5.07 ± 2.52	<0.001***

Table 2 : Comparison between 2 different times T1, T2 for G2 (control group)

Parameters	T1			T2		
	G1	G2	P	G1	G2	P
A- OLP (mm)	70.85±3.25	73.57±5.83	0.01*	71.79±3.35	75±5.9	0.003**
ANS-OLP (mm)	73.51±3.35	76.37±6.28	0.012*	74.35±3.36	77.99±6.28	0.002**
Pog- OLP (mm)	69.77±4.74	73.12±7.45	0.016*	73.03±4.6	74.76±7.62	0.211
Is- OLP (mm)	74.4±5.15	80.35±6.87	<0.001***	74.75±5.39	81.54±6.86	<0.001**
Ii- OLP (mm)	67.13±5.62	73.4±7.1	<0.001***	71.74±5.5	75.27±7.01	0.009**
Ms- OLP (mm)	34.92±3.69	37.75±5.05	0.003**	35.15±3.89	39.79±5.33	<0.001**
Mi- OLP (mm)	33.11±3.71	36.25±5.57	0.003**	37.5±3.87	39.11±5.44	0.118
Co- OLP(mm)	10.98±2.53	11.71±3.06	0.218	11.41±2.45	11.54±3.31	0.834
Ar- OLP (mm)	7.23±2.26	8.19±3.17	0.099	7.82±2.13	8.19±3.39	0.533
Mp- Ii(mm)	36.14±3.29	36.27±3.55	0.852	37.08±2.84	37.86±3.44	0.24
Mp-Mi(mm)	27.51±2.87	27.55±2.92	0.948	28.62±2.75	28.34±3.53	0.671
Mp- Ii (°)	97.05±5.88	96.39±7.54	0.65	99.03±6.06	97.79±7.38	0.394
Mp- Sn (°)	32.96±4.85	33.49±5.55	0.632	33.62±4.99	33.36±5.61	0.819
Mx- Is (mm)	26.01±2.82	25.59±3.33	0.516	27.97±2.85	27.2±3.12	0.224
Mx- Ms (mm)	17.5±2.91	17.69±2.04	0.731	18.12±2.84	19.29±2.41	0.041*
Na- ANS (mm)	45.66±3.04	47.17±6.63	0.034*	47.92±2.92	48.37±3.8	0.525
SN- PNS (mm)	38.88±2.99	39.92±3.36	0.121	40.29±2.88	40.5±3.36	0.75
ANS- Me (mm)	58.08±3.79	60.24±4.9	0.021*	59.97±3.75	61.72±4.85	0.056
Co- Pog (mm)	99.89±4.47	101.64±7.32	0.19	104.44±4.79	103.24±7.29	0.372
Overjet (mm)	7.27±2.04	6.95 ±2.65	0.532	2.66±2.19	5.07 ± 2.52	<0.001***

Table 3 : Comparison between groups G1 (treated group) and G2 (control group) at each time T1, T2.

	T2-T1		
Parameters	Δ **G1**	Δ **G2**	**P**
A- OLP (mm)	0.94±0.67	1.42±1.16	0.023**
ANS-OLP(mm)	0.84±0.78	1.61±1.38	0.003**
Pog- OLP (mm)	3.26±1.26	1.64±1.31	<0.001***
Is- OLP (mm)	0.35±1.68	1.19±2.52	0.063
Ii- OLP (mm)	4.61±1.59	1.87±1.23	<0.001***
Ms- OLP (mm)	0.23±1.15	2.03±1.3	<0.001***
Mi- OLP (mm)	4.39±1.38	2.86±2.16	<0.001***
Co- OLP (mm)	0.43±0.9	0.17±1.23	0.008**
Ar- OLP (mm)	0.59±0.85	0.00±1.33	0.013*
Mp- Ii (mm)	0.94±1.05	1.59±1.14	0.007**
Mp-Mi (mm)	1.11±0.84	0.79±1.73	0.251
Mp- Ii (°)	1.98±2.64	1.4±1.85	0.244
Mp- Sn (°)	0.66±1.58	0.12±1.25	0.012*
Mx- Is (mm)	1.96±0.99	1.61±0.86	0.081
Mx- Ms (mm)	0.62±0.71	1.6±0.95	<0.001***
Na- ANS (mm)	1.86±1.27	1.2±1.27	0.001**
SN- PNS (mm)	1.41±1.09	0.57±0.75	<0.001***
ANS- Me (mm)	1.89±1.33	1.49±1.03	0.121
Co- Pog (mm)	4.55±2.47	1.6±1.04	<0.001***
Overjet (mm)	4.61±1.59	1.87±1.228	<0.001***

Table 4 : Comparison in the changes (Δ) from T1 to T2 between groups G1 (treated group) and G2 (control group).

Parameters	Group 1			Group 2
	T1 to T2	T2 to T3	T1 to T3	T1 to T2
A- OLP (mm)	0.94 ± 0.67	1.32±1.32	2.22±1.15	1.42±1.16
ANS-OLP(mm)	0.84 ± 0.78	1.12±1.55	2.05±1.8	1.61±1.38
Pog- OLP (mm)	3.26 ±1.26	1.75±1.7	4.9±2.07	1.64±1.31
Is- OLP (mm)	0.35 ±1.68	0.6±2.28	1.43±3.52	1.19±2.52
Ii- OLP (mm)	4.61 ±1.59	0.87±2	5.8±2.06	1.87±1.23
Ms- OLP(mm)	0.23 ±1.15	2.1±2.67	2.22±3.04	2.03±1.3
Mi- OLP(mm)	4.39 ±1.38	1.87±3.06	6.45±3.43	2.86±2.16
Co- OLP(mm)	0.43 ±0.9	0.32±0.73	0.6±1.12	0.17±1.23
Ar- OLP(mm)	0.59±0.85	0.2±0.8	0.8±0.89	0.00±1.33
Mp- Ii(mm)	0.94±1.05	0.87±1.24	2.07±1.68	1.59±1.14
Mp-Mi(mm)	1.11±0.84	0.62±1.54	2.02±1.84	0.79±1.73
Mp- Ii (°)	1.98±2.64	-0.025±1.67	2.5±4.06	1.4±1.85
Mp- Sn (°)	0.66±1.58	-0.05±0.84	0.65±1.35	0.12±1.25
Mx- Is(mm)	1.96±0.99	0.52±0.85	2.5±1.45	1.61±0.86
Mx- Ms(mm)	0.62±0.71	1.15±1.31	1.7±1.2	1.6±0.95
Na- ANS(mm)	2.26±1.27	1.32±2.3	4.27±2.47	1.2±1.27
SN- PNS(mm)	1.41±1.09	0.97±1.85	2.52±2.35	0.57±0.75
ANS- Me(mm)	1.89±1.33	1.45±2	3.82±2.91	1.49±1.03
Co- Pog(mm)	4.55±2.47	3.1±2.25	8.85±3.96	1.6±1.04

Table 5 : Comparison for each groups G1 (treated group) and G2 (control group) at each time T1, T2, T3.

Table 6 : Correlation coefficient and significance for 19 parameters.

Parameter		DOLP A	DOLP ANS	DOLP PG1	DOLP IS	DOL II	DOLP MS	DOLP MI	DOLP CO	DOLP AR	DMp II	DMp MI	DMP II	DMD SN	DMX IS	DMX MS	DNA ANS	DSN PNS	DANS ME
DOLPANS	Pearson Correlation	0,272	1																
	Sig. (2-tailed)	0,055																	
DOLPPG1	Pearson Correlation	0,103	0,132	1															
	Sig. (2-tailed)	0,477	0,362																
DOLPIS	Pearson Correlation	0,0009	0,262	0,301	1														
	Sig. (2-tailed)	0,995	0,066	0,034															
DOLPII	Pearson Correlation	0,149	-0,018	0,485	0,384	1													
	Sig. (2-tailed)	0,303	0,899	0,0003	0,006														
DOLPMS	Pearson Correlation	0,229	0,025	0,212	0,087	0,699	1												
	Sig. (2-tailed)	0,110	0,864	0,139	0,548	0,006													
DOLPMI	Pearson Correlation	0,069	0,164	0,275	0,279	0,113	0,361	1											
	Sig. (2-tailed)	0,631	0,256	0,053	0,0499	0,436	0,0099												
DOLPCO	Pearson Correlation	0,094	-0,009	0,233	-0,027	0,005	0,065	-0,266	1										
	Sig. (2-tailed)	0,516	0,95	0,103	0,85	0,977	0,652	0,062											
DOLPAR	Pearson Correlation	-0,185	-0,093	-0,036	0,024	-0,251	0,051	-0,381	0,247	1									
	Sig. (2-tailed)	0,199	0,521	0,802	0,869	0,078	0,724	0,006	0,083										
DMpII	Pearson Correlation	0,316	0,025	0,219	0,089	0,246	-0,072	0,044	0,146	-0,045	1								
	Sig. (2-tailed)	0,025	0,862	0,127	0,537	0,085	0,617	0,759	0,312	0,758									
DMpMI	Pearson Correlation	0,074	0,306	0,016	0,098	0,074	0,005	0,189	0,01	0,098	0,253	1							
	Sig. (2-tailed)	0,608	0,031	0,914	0,499	0,609	0,973	0,187	0,943	0,496	0,077								
DMPII	Pearson Correlation	0,028	0,169	-0,044	0,448	0,253	-0,101	0,0413	0,018	-0,186	0,184	0,237	1						
	Sig. (2-tailed)	0,847	0,239	0,759	0,001	0,075	0,486	0,776	0,897	0,195	0,202	0,096							
DMDSN	Pearson Correlation	-0,024	-0,202	-0,018	0,065	0,011	-0,32	0,013	0,037	0,038	0,112	0,123	0,15	1					
	Sig. (2-tailed)	0,867	0,16	0,897	0,655	0,939	0,023	0,929	0,801	0,793	0,437	0,393	0,297						
DMXIS	Pearson Correlation	0,133	-0,114	0,094	-0,15	0,164	-0,188	-0,089	0,425	0,034	0,143	-0,0007	-0,004	0,149	1				
	Sig. (2-tailed)	0,356	0,431	0,515	0,298	0,255	0,189	0,539	0,002	0,813	0,321	0,996	0,977	0,299					
DMXMS	Pearson Correlation	0,302	0,164	-0,058	0,045	-0,084	-0,134	-0,095	0,021	-0,161	0,227	0,0877	0,31	0,127	0,028	1			
	Sig. (2-tailed)	0,033	0,254	0,687	0,755	0,562	0,352	0,509	0,883	0,265	0,113	0,544	0,378	0,844					
DNAANS	Pearson Correlation	0,239	0,379	0,072	0,155	0,051	0,109	0,332	-0,001	-0,036	0,396	0,453	0,1198	0,108	0,069	0,214	1		
	Sig. (2-tailed)	0,094	0,007	0,619	0,282	0,723	0,452	0,018	0,992	0,803	0,004	0,0009	0,411	0,453	0,633	0,136			
DSNPNS	Pearson Correlation	0,132	0,296	-0,031	-0,052	-0,009	-0,036	0,286	-0,017	-0,024	0,066	0,549	0,0313	0,201	0,109	0,146	0,533	1	
	Sig. (2-tailed)	0,362	0,041				0,803	0,044	0,906	0,868	0,647	3,6E-05	0,829	0,162	0,447	0,311	6,84E-05		
DANSME	Pearson Correlation	-0,047	0,218	-0,132	0,48	0,073	-0,209	0,206	-0,202	0,062	-0,055	0,155	0,437	0,239	-0,184	0,025	0,132	0,232	1
	Sig. (2-tailed)	0,745	0,128	0,364	0,0004	0,615	0,145	0,15	0,159	0,667	0,703	0,282	0,001	0,094	0,201	0,864	0,362	0,105	
DCOPG	Pearson Correlation	0,331	0,041	0,11	0,295	0,141	0,145	0,302	-0,06	-0,038	0,225	0,102	0,065	0,109	0,189	-0,0005	0,328	0,108	0,244
	Sig. (2-tailed)	0,019	0,776	0,445	0,038	0,328	0,024	0,865	0,329	0,677	0,792	0,481	0,655	0,448	0,187	0,997	0,02	0,455	0,088

%	Frequency	Valid percent	Cumulative Percent
-5.88	1	5.9	5.9
-5.56	1	5.9	11.8
0.00	4	23.5	35.3
2.56	1	5.9	41.2
5.88	1	5.9	47.1
7.69	1	5.9	52.9
11.11	1	5.9	58.8
14.29	4	23.5	82.4
18.92	1	5.9	88.2
20.00	1	5.9	94.1
25.00	1	5.9	100.00
TOTAL	17	100.00	

Table 7 : Frequencies table : Joint Space Index (JSI) for the left condyle at T1

%	Frequency	Valid percent	Cumulative Percent
-20.00	1	5.9	5.9
-11.11	1	5.9	11.8
-7.69	1	5.9	17.6
-4.76	1	5.9	23.5
-3.45	1	5.9	29.4
0.00	3	17.6	47.1
4.76	1	5.9	52.9
5.26	2	11.8	64.7
7.14	1	5.9	70.6
8.11	1	5.9	76.5
11.11	1	5.9	82.4
14.29	2	11.8	94.1
16.67	1	5.9	100.00
TOTAL	17	100.00	

Table 8 : Frequencies table : Joint Space Index (JSI) for the right condyle at T1

%	Frequency	Valid percent	Cumulative Percent
-4.76	1	5.9	5.9
0.00	7	41.2	47.1
4.35	1	5.9	52.9
5.26	1	5.9	58.8
5.88	1	5.9	64.7
9.09	1	5.9	70.6
11.11	1	5.9	76.5
20.00	2	11.8	88.2
28.00	1	5.9	94.1
33.00	1	5.9	100.00
TOTAL	17	100.00	

Table 9 : Frequencies table : Joint Space Index (JSI) for the left condyle at T2

%	Frequency	Valid percent	Cumulative Percent
-7.94	1	5.9	5.9
-6.67	1	5.9	11.8
-5.26	1	5.9	17.6
-4.35	1	5.9	23.5
0.00	4	23.5	47.1
6.25	1	5.9	52.9
6.67	1	5.9	58.8
7.69	1	5.9	64.7
11.11	3	17.7	82.4
13.73	1	5.9	88.2
14.29	2	11.8	100.00
TOTAL	17	100.00	

Table 10 : Frequencies table : Joint Space Index (JSI) for the right condyle at T2

%	Frequency	Valid percent	Cumulative Percent
-20.00	1	5.9	5.9
-18.92	1	5.9	11.8
-14.29	2	11.8	23.5
-5.88	1	5.9	29.4
-5.23	1	5.9	35.3
-4.76	1	5.9	41.2
0.00	1	5.9	47.1
1.40	1	5.9	52.9
4.35	1	5.9	58.8
5.26	1	5.9	64.7
5.71	2	11.8	76.5
5.88	1	5.9	82.4
8.33	1	5.9	88.2
16.67	1	5.9	94.1
25.44	1	5.9	100.0
TOTAL	17	100	

Table 11 : Frequencies table : Differences between the Joint Space Index (ΔJSI) for the left condyle (T2 – T1)

%	Frequency	Valid percent	Cumulative Percent
-10.53	1	5.9	5.9
-7.14	1	5.9	11.8
-6.67	1	5.9	17.6
-4.76	1	5.9	23.5
-4.44	1	5.9	29.4
-3.69	1	5.9	35.3
-3.17	1	5.9	41.2
-2.94	1	5.9	47.1
-1.86	1	5.9	52.9
0.00	1	5.9	58.8
3.34	1	5.9	64.7
4.76	1	5.9	70.6
5.85	1	5.9	76.5
11.11	1	5.9	82.4
11.11	1	5.9	88.2
14.29	1	5.9	94.1
27.69	1	5.9	100.0
TOTAL	17	100.0	

Table 12 : Frequencies table : Differences between the Joint Space Index (ΔJSI) for the right condyle (T2 – T1)

References

1. Jakobsson S O. Cephalometric evaluation of treatment effect on Class II Division 1 malocclusion. Am J Orthod. 1967; 53: 446-457.

2. Harvold E, Vargervik K. Morphogenetic response to activator treatment. Am J Orthod. 1971; 60: 478-490.

3. Pancherz H. The Herbst appliance – its biological effects and clinical use. Am J Orthod. 1985; 87: 1-20.

4. Pancherz H. The mechanism of Class II correction in Herbst appliance treatment. Am J Orthod. 1982; 82: 104-113.

5. Herbst E. Dreissigjährige Erfahrungen mit dem Retentions Scharnier. Zahnärztl Rundschau. 1934; 43: 1515-1524, 1563-1568, 1611-1616.

6. Pancherz H. Treatment of Class II malocclusions by bite jumping with the Herbst appliance: a cephalometric investigation. Am J Orthod. 1979; 76: 423-441.

7. Pancherz H. The effect of continuous bite jumping on the dentofacial complex: a follow-up study after Herbst appliance treatment of Class II malocclusions. Europ J Orthod. 1981; 3: 49-60.

8. Pancherz H, Malmgren O, Hägg U, Ömblus J. & Hansen K. Class II Correction in Herbst and Bass Therapy. A comparative study considering somatic maturity and skeletofacial morphology. Europ J Orthod. 1989, 11: 17-30.

9. Pancherz H. Vertical dentofacial changes during Herbst appliance treatment: a cephalometric investigation. Swed Dent J Supp. 1982; 15: 189-196.

10. Sarnäs K, Pancherz H, Rune B, Selvik G. Hemifacial microsomia treated with the Herbst appliance: report of a case analyzed by means of roentgen stereometry and metallic implants. Am J Orthod. 1982: 85: 68-74.

11. Rogers M.B. Herbst Appliance Variations. J Clin Orthod. 2003; 37 (3) : 156-161.

12. Hashim H.A. Analysis of activator treatment changes. Austr Orthod J. 1991; 12: 100-104.

13. Petrovic A.G, Stutzmann J, Outdet C. Control processes in the postnatal growth of the mandibular condylar cartilage in: McNamara

J.A.ed. Determinants of mandibular form and growth. Monograph 4. Craniofacial Growth Series. Ann Arbor: Center of Human Growth and Development University of Michigan, 1975: 101-153.

14. Aelbers C.M.F. Orthopedics in orthodontics. Part I, fiction or reality—a review of the literature. Am J Orthod Dentofac Orthop. 1996; 110: 513-519.

15. Woodside D.G, Hetaxas A, Alluna G. The influence of functional appliance therapy on glenoid fossa remodeling. Am J Orthod Dentofac Orthop. 1987; 92: 181-198.

16. Wieslander L. Long-term effect of treatment with the headgear-Herbst appliance in the early mixed dentition. Stability or relapse?. Am J Orthod Dentofac Orthop. 1993; 104: 319-329.

17. Ruf S, Pancherz H. Temporomandibular joint growth adaptation in Herbst treatment: a prospective magnetic resonance imaging and cephalometric roentgenographic study. Europ J Orthod. 1998; 20: 375-388.

18. Paulsen H.U, Karle A, Bakke M, Herskind A. CT scanning and radiographic analysis of temporomandibular joints and cephalometric analysis in a case of herbst treatment in late puberty. Europ J Orthod. 1995; 17: 165-175.

19. Paulsen H.U, Karle A. Computer tomographic and radiologic changes in the temporomandibular joints of two young adults with occlusal asymmetry, treated with the Herbst appliance. Europ J Orthod. 2000; 22: 649-656.

20. Dermaut L.R, Aelbers C.M.F. Orthopedics in orthodontics: Fiction or reality: A review of the literature, Part II. Am J Orthod Dentofac Orthop. 1996; 110: 667-671.

21. Popowich K, Nebbe B, Paul W. Effect of Herbst treatment on temporomandibular joint morphology: A systematic literature review. Am J Orthod Dentofac Orthop. 2003; 123: 388-394.

22. Pruvost J.L. The modular Palatal Disjunctor Appliance. J Clin Orthod. 1989; 23: 36-40.

23. Dischinger T. Edgewise Herbst Appliance. J Clin Orthod. 1995; 29: 738-742.

24. Kamelchuk L, Grace M, Major P. Post imaging Temporomandibular Joint Space Analysis. Journal of Craniomandibular practice. 1996; 26: 23-29.

25. Pangrazio-Kulbersh V, Berger J.L. Comparison of treatment of identical twins. Am J Orthod Dentofac Orthop. 1993; 103: 131–137.

26. Croft R.S , Buschang P.H , English J, Meyer R. A cephalometric and tomographic evaluation of Herbst treatment in the mixed dentition. Am J Orthod Dentofac Orthop. 1999; 116: 435-443.

27. Falck F, Fränkel R. Clinical relevance of step-by-step mandibular advancement in the treatment of mandibular retrusion using the Frankel appliance. Am J Orthod Dentofac Orthop 1989; 96: 333-341..

28. Hansen K, Pancherz H, Hagg U. Long term effects of the Herbst appliance in relation to the treatment growth period: a cephalometric study. Europ J Orthod. 1991; 13: 471-481.

29. Pancherz H, Hägg U. Dentofacial orthopedics in relation to somatic maturation. Am J Orthod. 1985; 88: 273-287.

30. Pancherz H, The Head Gear effect of the Herbst appliance : a cephalometric long term study. Am J Orthod Dentofac Orthop. 1993; 103: 510-520.

31. Valant J.R, Sinclair P.M. Treatment effects of Herbst appliance. Am J Orthod Dentofac Orthop. 1989; 95: 138-147.

32. Graf E.J. Funktionelle Kräfte bei bimaxillären Regulationsapparaten [Thesis]. Universität Bern, 1962.

33. Witt E, Komposch G. Intermaxilläre Kraftwirkung bimaxillärer Geräte. Fortschr Kieferorthop 1971; 32: 345-352.

34. Mills J.R.E. Clinical control of craniofacial growth: a skeptic's viewpoint. In: McNamara JA Jr, Ribbens KA, Howe RP, eds. Clinical alteration of the growing face. Monograph 14, Craniofacial Growth Series, Ann Arbor, Michigan: Center for Human Growth and Development, University of Michigan, 1983: 17-39.

35. Pancherz H. Class ll relapse after Herbst treatment, Am J Orthod Dentofac Orthop. 1991; 100 : 220-233.

36. Obijou C, Pancherz H. Herbst appliance treatment of Class II, Division 2 malocclusions. Am J Orthod Dentofac Orthop. 1997; 112: 287-291.

37. Pancherz H, Hansen K. Occlusal changes during and after Herbst treatment: a cephalometric investigation. Eur J Orthod. 1986; 8: 215-228.

38. Pancherz H, Weschler D. Efficiency of three mandibular anchorage forms in Herbst treatment: a cephalometric investigation. Angle Orthod. 2005; 75(1): 23-27.

39. Konik M, Pancherz H, Hansen K. The mechanism of Class II correction in late Herbst treatment. Am J Orthod Dentofac Orthop. 1997; 112: 87-91.

40. Pancherz H, Anehus-Pancherz M. Headgear effect of the Herbst appliance. Am J Orthod Dentofac Orthop. 1993; 103: 510–520.

41. Ruf S, Pancherz H. The effect of Herbst appliance treatment on the mandibular plane angle: A cephalometric roentgenographic study. Am J Orthod Dentofac Orthop. 1996; 110: 225–229.

42. Vardimon A, Koklu S, Iseri H, Shpack N, Frickee J, Mete L. An assessment of skeletal and dental responses to the functional magnetic system. Am J Orthod Dentofac Orthop. 2001; 120: 416-426.

43. Adenwalla S, Kronman J, Attarzadeh F. Porion and condyle as cephalometric landmarks. Am J Orthod Dentofac Orthop. 1988; 94: 411–415.

44. Fischer S, Pancherz H. Amount and direction of temporomandibular joint growth changes in Herbst treatment: a cephalometric long-term investigation. Angle Orthod. 2003; 73(5): 493-501.

45. Pancherz H, Michailidou C. Temporomandibular joint growth changes in hyperdivergent and hypodivergent Herbst subjects. A long-term roentgenographic cephalometric study. Am J Orthod Dentofac Orthop. 2004; 126 (2): 153-161; quiz 254-255.

46. Kohlas P, Ruf S, Pancherz H. Effective condylar growth and chin position changes in Herbst treatment : A cephalometric roentgenographic long-term study. Am J Orthod Dentofac Orthop. 1998; 114: 437-446.

47. Voudouris J.C, Kuftinec M.M. Improved clinical use of Twin-block and Herbst as a result of radiating viscoelastic tissue forces on the condyle and fossa in treatment and long-term retention: Growth relativity. Am J Orthod Dentofac Orthop. 2000; 117(3): 247-266.

48. Voudouris J.C, Woodside D.G, Altuna G, Angelopoulos G, Bourque P.J, Lacouture C.Y. Condyle-fossa modifications and muscle interactions during Herbst treatment, Part 2. Results and conclusions. Am J Orthod Dentofac Orthop. 2003; 124(1): 13-29.

49. Buschang P.H, Santos-Pinto A. Condylar growth and glenoid fossa displacement during childhood and adolescence. Am J Orthod Dentofac Orthop. 1998; 113(4): 437-442.

50. McNamara J, Hinton R, Hoffman D. Histologic analysis of temporomandibular joint adaptation to protrusive function in young adult Rhesus monkeys. Am J Orthod. 1982; 82: 288-298.

51. Woodside D.G, Metaxas A, Altuna G. The influence of functional appliance therapy on glenoid fossa remodeling. Am J Orthod Dentofac Orthop. 1987; 92: 181-198.

52. Guner A, Ozturk Y, Sayman H. Evaluation of the effects of functional orthopaedic treatment on temporomandibular joints with single-photon emission computerized tomography. Europ J Orthod. 2003; 25: 9-12.

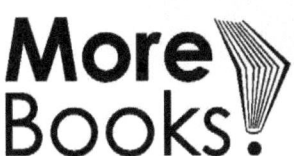
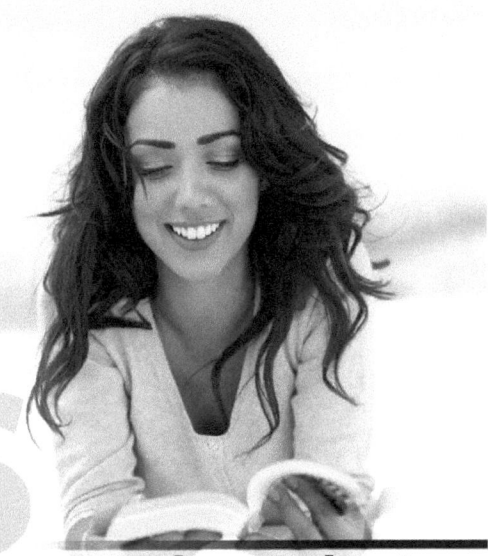
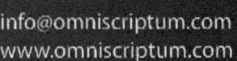
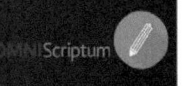

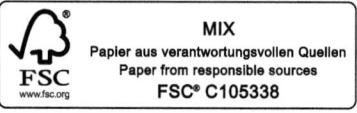

Printed by Books on Demand GmbH, Norderstedt / Germany